Inspirational Weight Loss

Daily Quotes to Lose Weight By

CW01497755

By Josephina Protopappas

Inspirational Weight Loss
Daily Quotes to Lose Weight By

Printed in the United States of America

Dedication

This book is dedicated to those who struggle with their weight. May we all end the struggle and find new ways to live our lives lovingly in our own bodies so we can have a little more peace, a little more joy and a lot less weight! ❤

How to use this book!

Do you worry about your weight, and shedding the pounds? Do you wonder if you look good or not; feel healthy or not? Then this little book is for you! It is a gentle, daily way to look at yourself and find better ways to address your weight - quietly, consistently and with self-compassion. These quotes give you a little something to give yourself everyday while you are on your journey to weight loss.

Find the gift in each quote. You can read a quote a day, or you can read one every other day, skip around the book, or however you wish to do it - just do it!

At any time of the day, read a quote. Think about it for just a few seconds. Take a few more seconds to think about *how you will* incorporate the quote into your life for the day, as it applies to your weight, or any other part of your life.

And, at the end of your day, before you settle in for a good night's sleep, there is a place in your book to journal how the quote helped you in its quiet, gentle way. Notice what your thoughts were, and how your behavior may have changed. Then, smile, and give thanks for your life and whatever else you want to give thanks and gratitude.

The most important part is that you enjoy yourself. Give yourself those little bits of time each day, to look at your life through a simple little quote. Enjoy!

- Josephina

Let's begin.

"Experience a little bit of better everyday and watch your life change!"

— Josephina!

Beginning Your Day

What does this quote mean to me personally today?

_____

_____

_____

How will I apply this quote today?

_____

_____

_____

Who else needs to hear this quote today?

_____

_____

_____

At the End of Your Day

How did I apply this quote today?

_____

_____

_____

What will I do differently going forward?

_____

_____

_____

"Our deepest fear is not that we are inadequate. It is that we are powerful beyond our measure. It is our light, not our darkness that most frightens us. We ask ourselves, 'Who am I to be brilliant, gorgeous, talented, fabulous?' Actually, who are you not to be? Your playing small does not serve the world. There is nothing enlightened about shrinking so that other people won't feel insecure around you."   *–Marianne Williamson*

Beginning Your Day
What does this quote mean to me personally today?

_____

_____

_____

How will I apply this quote today?

_____

_____

_____

Who else needs to hear this quote today?

_____

_____

_____

At the End of Your Day
How did I apply this quote today?

_____

_____

_____

What will I do differently going forward?

_____

_____

_____

"The most beautiful people are those who have known defeat, known suffering, known struggle, known loss, and have found their way out of the depths. These persons have an appreciation, a sensitivity, and an understanding of life that fills them with compassion, gentleness, and a deep loving concern. Beautiful people do not just happen."   *—Elizabeth Kubler Ross*

Beginning Your Day
What does this quote mean to me personally today?

_____

_____

How will I apply this quote today?

_____

_____

Who else needs to hear this quote today?

_____

_____

_____

At the End of Your Day
How did I apply this quote today?

_____

_____

What will I do differently going forward?

_____

_____

_____

"Be thankful for what you have; you'll end up having more. If you concentrate on what you don't have, you will never, ever have enough."

–Oprah Winfrey

Beginning Your Day
What does this quote mean to me personally today?

_____

_____

How will I apply this quote today?

_____

_____

Who else needs to hear this quote today?

_____

_____

_____

At the End of Your Day
How did I apply this quote today?

_____

_____

What will I do differently going forward?

_____

_____

_____

"Believe you can and you're half way there."

—Theodore Roosevelt

Beginning Your Day
What does this quote mean to me personally today?

_____

_____

_____

How will I apply this quote today?

_____

_____

_____

Who else needs to hear this quote today?

_____

_____

_____

At the End of Your Day
How did I apply this quote today?

_____

_____

_____

What will I do differently going forward?

_____

_____

_____

_____

"Thousands of candles can be lighted from a single candle, and the life of that candle will not be shortened. Happiness never decreases by being shared."

—Buddha

Beginning Your Day
What does this quote mean to me personally today?

_____

_____

_____

How will I apply this quote today?

_____

_____

_____

Who else needs to hear this quote today?

_____

_____

_____

At the End of Your Day
How did I apply this quote today?

_____

_____

What will I do differently going forward?

_____

_____

_____

"You can never cross the ocean until you have the courage to lose sight of the shore."

—Christopher Columbus

Beginning Your Day

What does this quote mean to me personally today?

_____

_____

_____

How will I apply this quote today?

_____

_____

_____

Who else needs to hear this quote today?

_____

_____

_____

At the End of Your Day

How did I apply this quote today?

_____

_____

_____

What will I do differently going forward?

_____

_____

_____

"If it isn't making you better, it isn't love. True love makes you more of who you are, not less."

–Mandy Hale

Beginning Your Day
What does this quote mean to me personally today?

_____

_____

How will I apply this quote today?

_____

_____

Who else needs to hear this quote today?

_____

_____

_____

At the End of Your Day
How did I apply this quote today?

_____

_____

What will I do differently going forward?

_____

_____

_____

"If you accept the expectations of others, especially negative ones, then you never will change the outcome."

—Michael Jordan

Beginning Your Day
What does this quote mean to me personally today?

_____

_____

_____

How will I apply this quote today?

_____

_____

_____

Who else needs to hear this quote today?

_____

_____

_____

At the End of Your Day
How did I apply this quote today?

_____

_____

_____

What will I do differently going forward?

_____

_____

_____

_____

"If we did all the things we are capable of, we would literally astound ourselves."

–Thomas A. Edison

Beginning Your Day
What does this quote mean to me personally today?

_____

_____

_____

How will I apply this quote today?

_____

_____

_____

Who else needs to hear this quote today?

_____

_____

_____

At the End of Your Day
How did I apply this quote today?

_____

_____

_____

What will I do differently going forward?

_____

_____

_____

"The minute you start compromising for the sake of massaging somebody's ego, that's it, game over."

–Gordon Ramsay

Beginning Your Day
What does this quote mean to me personally today?

_____

_____

_____

How will I apply this quote today?

_____

_____

_____

Who else needs to hear this quote today?

_____

_____

_____

At the End of Your Day
How did I apply this quote today?

_____

_____

_____

What will I do differently going forward?

_____

_____

_____

_____

"Look up at the stars and not down at your feet.
Try to make sense of what you see, and wonder
about what makes the universe exist. Be curious."

–*Stephen Hawking*

Beginning Your Day
What does this quote mean to me personally today?

_____

_____

How will I apply this quote today?

_____

_____

Who else needs to hear this quote today?

_____

_____

_____

At the End of Your Day
How did I apply this quote today?

_____

_____

What will I do differently going forward?

_____

_____

_____

"Our ambition should be to rule ourselves, the true kingdom for each one of us; and true progress is to know more, and be more, and to do more."

–Oscar Wilde

Beginning Your Day
What does this quote mean to me personally today?

_____

_____

_____

How will I apply this quote today?

_____

_____

_____

Who else needs to hear this quote today?

_____

_____

_____

At the End of Your Day
How did I apply this quote today?

_____

_____

_____

What will I do differently going forward?

_____

_____

_____

_____

"You miss 100% of the shots you don't take."

–Wayne Gretzky

Beginning Your Day
What does this quote mean to me personally today?

_____

_____

How will I apply this quote today?

_____

_____

Who else needs to hear this quote today?

_____

_____

_____

At the End of Your Day
How did I apply this quote today?

_____

_____

What will I do differently going forward?

_____

_____

_____

"If you really want to do something, you will find a way. If you don't, you'll find an excuse."

–Jim Rohn

Beginning Your Day
What does this quote mean to me personally today?

_____

_____

_____

How will I apply this quote today?

_____

_____

_____

Who else needs to hear this quote today?

_____

_____

_____

At the End of Your Day
How did I apply this quote today?

_____

_____

_____

What will I do differently going forward?

_____

_____

_____

"I like nonsense, it wakes up the brain cells.
Fantasy is a necessary ingredient in living, it's a
way of looking at life through the wrong end of a
telescope. Which is what I do, and that enables
you to laugh at life's realities."

–Dr. Seuss

Beginning Your Day
What does this quote mean to me personally today?

_____

_____

How will I apply this quote today?

_____

_____

Who else needs to hear this quote today?

_____

_____

_____

At the End of Your Day
How did I apply this quote today?

_____

_____

What will I do differently going forward?

_____

_____

_____

"Carry out a random act of kindness, with no expectation of reward, safe in the knowledge that one day someone might do the same for you."

–Princess Diana

Beginning Your Day
What does this quote mean to me personally today?

_____
_____
_____

How will I apply this quote today?

_____
_____
_____

Who else needs to hear this quote today?

_____
_____
_____

At the End of Your Day
How did I apply this quote today?

_____
_____
_____

What will I do differently going forward?

_____
_____
_____
_____

"Success is not final, failure is not fatal; it is courage to continue that counts."

–Winston Churchill

Beginning Your Day
What does this quote mean to me personally today?

_____

_____

_____

How will I apply this quote today?

_____

_____

_____

Who else needs to hear this quote today?

_____

_____

_____

At the End of Your Day
How did I apply this quote today?

_____

_____

_____

What will I do differently going forward?

_____

_____

_____

"If you were born poor it's not your mistake, but if you die poor, it is your mistake."

—Bill Gates

Beginning Your Day
What does this quote mean to me personally today?

_____

_____

_____

How will I apply this quote today?

_____

_____

_____

Who else needs to hear this quote today?

_____

_____

_____

At the End of Your Day
How did I apply this quote today?

_____

_____

_____

What will I do differently going forward?

_____

_____

_____

_____

"A seed planted in the ground does not feel its lack of roots, stem and petals as a 'weakness' or being 'less than'. It simply sees an opportunity to grow and then does."

–Michael Stevenson

Beginning Your Day
What does this quote mean to me personally today?

_____

_____

How will I apply this quote today?

_____

_____

Who else needs to hear this quote today?

_____

_____

_____

At the End of Your Day
How did I apply this quote today?

_____

_____

What will I do differently going forward?

_____

_____

_____

"Being rich is a good thing. Not just in the obvious sense of benefitting you and your family, but in the broader sense. Profits are not a zero sum game. The more you make, the more of a financial impact you can have."

—Mark Cuban

Beginning Your Day
What does this quote mean to me personally today?

_____

_____

How will I apply this quote today?

_____

_____

Who else needs to hear this quote today?

_____

_____

_____

At the End of Your Day
How did I apply this quote today?

_____

_____

What will I do differently going forward?

_____

_____

_____

"People say I make strange choices, but they're not strange for me. My sickness is that I'm fascinated by human behaviour, by what's underneath the surface, by the worlds inside people."

–Johnny Depp

Beginning Your Day
What does this quote mean to me personally today?

_____

_____

How will I apply this quote today?

_____

_____

Who else needs to hear this quote today?

_____

_____

_____

At the End of Your Day
How did I apply this quote today?

_____

_____

What will I do differently going forward?

_____

_____

_____

"Leadership is getting players to believe in you. If you tell a teammate you're ready to play as tough as you're able to, you'd better go out there and do it. Players will see right through a phony, and they can tell when you're not giving it all you've got."

–Larry Bird

Beginning Your Day
What does this quote mean to me personally today?

_____

_____

How will I apply this quote today?

_____

_____

Who else needs to hear this quote today?

_____

_____

_____

At the End of Your Day
How did I apply this quote today?

_____

_____

What will I do differently going forward?

_____

_____

_____

"When saying 'yes' to others, make sure you aren't saying 'no' to yourself."

–Paulo Coehlo

Beginning Your Day
What does this quote mean to me personally today?

_____

_____

_____

How will I apply this quote today?

_____

_____

_____

Who else needs to hear this quote today?

_____

_____

_____

At the End of Your Day
How did I apply this quote today?

_____

_____

_____

What will I do differently going forward?

_____

_____

_____

"I attribute my success to this: I never gave or took any excuse."

–Florence Nightingale

Beginning Your Day
What does this quote mean to me personally today?

_____

_____

How will I apply this quote today?

_____

_____

Who else needs to hear this quote today?

_____

_____

_____

At the End of Your Day
How did I apply this quote today?

_____

_____

What will I do differently going forward?

_____

_____

_____

"I can't change the direction of the wind, but I can adjust my sails to always reach my destination."

–Jimmy Dean

Beginning Your Day
What does this quote mean to me personally today?

_____

_____

_____

How will I apply this quote today?

_____

_____

_____

Who else needs to hear this quote today?

_____

_____

_____

At the End of Your Day
How did I apply this quote today?

_____

_____

_____

What will I do differently going forward?

_____

_____

_____

"Strong minds discuss ideas, average minds discuss events, weak minds discuss people."

–Socrates

Beginning Your Day
What does this quote mean to me personally today?

_____

_____

_____

How will I apply this quote today?

_____

_____

_____

Who else needs to hear this quote today?

_____

_____

_____

At the End of Your Day
How did I apply this quote today?

_____

_____

_____

What will I do differently going forward?

_____

_____

_____

"Let us always meet each other with a smile, for the smile is the beginning of love."

–Mother Teresa

Beginning Your Day
What does this quote mean to me personally today?

_____

_____

How will I apply this quote today?

_____

_____

Who else needs to hear this quote today?

_____

_____

_____

At the End of Your Day
How did I apply this quote today?

_____

_____

What will I do differently going forward?

_____

_____

_____

"Tell me and I forget. Teach me and I remember. Involve me and I learn."

–Benjamin Franklin

Beginning Your Day
What does this quote mean to me personally today?

_____
_____
_____

How will I apply this quote today?

_____
_____
_____

Who else needs to hear this quote today?

_____
_____
_____

At the End of Your Day
How did I apply this quote today?

_____
_____
_____

What will I do differently going forward?

_____
_____
_____
_____

"Your journey has molded you for your greater good, and it was exactly what it needed to be. Don't think that you've lost time. It took each and every situation you have encountered to bring you to the now. And now is right on time."

–Asha Tyson

Beginning Your Day
What does this quote mean to me personally today?

_____

_____

How will I apply this quote today?

_____

_____

Who else needs to hear this quote today?

_____

_____

_____

At the End of Your Day
How did I apply this quote today?

_____

_____

What will I do differently going forward?

_____

_____

_____

"I want everybody to be happier. I would love for the world to be happier. I think it's our one thing that we all share. We focus so much on our differences, and that is creating, I think, a lot of chaos and negativity and bullying in the world. And I think everybody should focus on what we all have in common, which is, we all want to be happy." —*Ellen DeGeneres*

Beginning Your Day
What does this quote mean to me personally today?

_____

_____

_____

How will I apply this quote today?

_____

_____

_____

Who else needs to hear this quote today?

_____

_____

_____

At the End of Your Day
How did I apply this quote today?

_____

_____

_____

What will I do differently going forward?

_____

_____

_____

"You can't have a better tomorrow if you are always thinking about yesterday."

–Charles F. Kettering

Beginning Your Day
What does this quote mean to me personally today?

_____

_____

How will I apply this quote today?

_____

_____

Who else needs to hear this quote today?

_____

_____

_____

At the End of Your Day
How did I apply this quote today?

_____

_____

What will I do differently going forward?

_____

_____

_____

"Be grateful for what you have and stop complaining. It bores everyone else, does you no good, and doesn't solve any problems."

–Zig Ziglar

Beginning Your Day
What does this quote mean to me personally today?

_____

_____

_____

How will I apply this quote today?

_____

_____

_____

Who else needs to hear this quote today?

_____

_____

_____

At the End of Your Day
How did I apply this quote today?

_____

_____

_____

What will I do differently going forward?

_____

_____

_____

"Live as if you were to die tomorrow. Learn as if you were to live forever."

—Mahatma Gandhi

Beginning Your Day
What does this quote mean to me personally today?

_____
_____
_____

How will I apply this quote today?

_____
_____
_____

Who else needs to hear this quote today?

_____
_____
_____

At the End of Your Day
How did I apply this quote today?

_____
_____

What will I do differently going forward?

_____
_____
_____

"Prosperity is your ability to trust that the divine will provide and replenish."

—*Glenn Morshower*

Beginning Your Day
What does this quote mean to me personally today?

_____

_____

_____

How will I apply this quote today?

_____

_____

_____

Who else needs to hear this quote today?

_____

_____

_____

At the End of Your Day
How did I apply this quote today?

_____

_____

_____

What will I do differently going forward?

_____

_____

_____

_____

"If it scares you, it might be a good thing to try."

–Seth Godin

Beginning Your Day
What does this quote mean to me personally today?

_____

_____

How will I apply this quote today?

_____

_____

Who else needs to hear this quote today?

_____

_____

At the End of Your Day
How did I apply this quote today?

_____

_____

What will I do differently going forward?

_____

_____

_____

"The measure of who we are is what we do with what we have."

–Vince Lombardi

Beginning Your Day
What does this quote mean to me personally today?

_____

_____

_____

How will I apply this quote today?

_____

_____

_____

Who else needs to hear this quote today?

_____

_____

_____

At the End of Your Day
How did I apply this quote today?

_____

_____

_____

What will I do differently going forward?

_____

_____

_____

_____

"Our minds influence the key activity of the brain, which then influences everything; perception, cognition, thoughts and feelings, personal relationships; they're all a projection of you."

–Deepak Chopra

Beginning Your Day
What does this quote mean to me personally today?

_____

_____

_____

How will I apply this quote today?

_____

_____

_____

Who else needs to hear this quote today?

_____

_____

_____

At the End of Your Day
How did I apply this quote today?

_____

_____

_____

What will I do differently going forward?

_____

_____

_____

"Strive not to be a success, but rather to be of value."

–Albert Einstein

Beginning Your Day

What does this quote mean to me personally today?

_____

_____

_____

How will I apply this quote today?

_____

_____

_____

Who else needs to hear this quote today?

_____

_____

_____

At the End of Your Day

How did I apply this quote today?

_____

_____

_____

What will I do differently going forward?

_____

_____

_____

"There is little success where there is little laughter."

–Andrew Carnegie

Beginning Your Day
What does this quote mean to me personally today?

_____

_____

How will I apply this quote today?

_____

_____

Who else needs to hear this quote today?

_____

_____

_____

At the End of Your Day
How did I apply this quote today?

_____

_____

What will I do differently going forward?

_____

_____

_____

"If you hear a voice within you say 'you cannot paint,' then by all means, paint, and that voice will be silenced."

–Vincent Van Gogh

Beginning Your Day
What does this quote mean to me personally today?

_____
_____
_____

How will I apply this quote today?

_____
_____
_____

Who else needs to hear this quote today?

_____
_____
_____

At the End of Your Day
How did I apply this quote today?

_____
_____
_____

What will I do differently going forward?

_____
_____
_____

"Money and success don't change people; they merely amplify what is already there."

—Will Smith

Beginning Your Day
What does this quote mean to me personally today?

_____

_____

How will I apply this quote today?

_____

_____

Who else needs to hear this quote today?

_____

_____

_____

At the End of Your Day
How did I apply this quote today?

_____

_____

What will I do differently going forward?

_____

_____

_____

"I'd rather regret the things I've done, than regret the things I haven't done."

–Lucille Ball

Beginning Your Day
What does this quote mean to me personally today?

_____

_____

_____

How will I apply this quote today?

_____

_____

_____

Who else needs to hear this quote today?

_____

_____

_____

At the End of Your Day
How did I apply this quote today?

_____

_____

_____

What will I do differently going forward?

_____

_____

_____

"Don't let the fear of striking out hold you back."

–Babe Ruth

Beginning Your Day
What does this quote mean to me personally today?

_____

_____

How will I apply this quote today?

_____

_____

Who else needs to hear this quote today?

_____

_____

At the End of Your Day
How did I apply this quote today?

_____

_____

What will I do differently going forward?

_____

_____

_____

"Listen to the mustn'ts, child. Listen to the don'ts. Listen to the shouldn'ts, the impossibles, the won'ts. Listen to the never haves, THEN listen close to me... Anything can happen, child. Anything can be."

–Shel Silverstein

Beginning Your Day
What does this quote mean to me personally today?

_____

_____

How will I apply this quote today?

_____

_____

Who else needs to hear this quote today?

_____

_____

_____

At the End of Your Day
How did I apply this quote today?

_____

_____

What will I do differently going forward?

_____

_____

_____

"Happiness is not something you postpone for the future; it is something you design for the present."

—Jim Rohn

Beginning Your Day
What does this quote mean to me personally today?

_____
_____
_____

How will I apply this quote today?

_____
_____
_____

Who else needs to hear this quote today?

_____
_____
_____

At the End of Your Day
How did I apply this quote today?

_____
_____
_____

What will I do differently going forward?

_____
_____
_____

"Never make someone a priority when all you are to them is an option."

–Maya Angelou

Beginning Your Day
What does this quote mean to me personally today?

_____

_____

_____

How will I apply this quote today?

_____

_____

_____

Who else needs to hear this quote today?

_____

_____

_____

At the End of Your Day
How did I apply this quote today?

_____

_____

_____

What will I do differently going forward?

_____

_____

_____

"The only way to permanently change the temperature in the room is to reset the thermostat. In the same way, the only way to change your level of financial success 'permanently' is to reset your financial thermostat. But it is your choice whether you choose to change."

— *T. Harv Eker*

Beginning Your Day
What does this quote mean to me personally today?

_____

_____

How will I apply this quote today?

_____

_____

Who else needs to hear this quote today?

_____

_____

At the End of Your Day
How did I apply this quote today?

_____

_____

What will I do differently going forward?

_____

_____

_____

"Be yourself; everyone else is already taken."

–Oscar Wilde

Beginning Your Day
What does this quote mean to me personally today?

_____

_____

_____

How will I apply this quote today?

_____

_____

_____

Who else needs to hear this quote today?

_____

_____

_____

At the End of Your Day
How did I apply this quote today?

_____

_____

_____

What will I do differently going forward?

_____

_____

_____

_____

"A successful man will profit from his mistakes and try again in a different way."

–Dale Carnegie

Beginning Your Day
What does this quote mean to me personally today?

_____

_____

_____

How will I apply this quote today?

_____

_____

_____

Who else needs to hear this quote today?

_____

_____

_____

At the End of Your Day
How did I apply this quote today?

_____

_____

_____

What will I do differently going forward?

_____

_____

_____

"Communication is a skill that you can learn. It's like riding a bicycle or typing. If you're willing to work at it, you can rapidly improve the quality of every part of your life."

—Brian Tracy

Beginning Your Day
What does this quote mean to me personally today?

_____

_____

_____

How will I apply this quote today?

_____

_____

_____

Who else needs to hear this quote today?

_____

_____

_____

At the End of Your Day
How did I apply this quote today?

_____

_____

_____

What will I do differently going forward?

_____

_____

_____

"I do not fix problems. I fix my thinking. The problems fix themselves."

–Louise Hay

Beginning Your Day
What does this quote mean to me personally today?

_____

_____

_____

How will I apply this quote today?

_____

_____

_____

Who else needs to hear this quote today?

_____

_____

_____

At the End of Your Day
How did I apply this quote today?

_____

_____

What will I do differently going forward?

_____

_____

_____

"Progress is impossible without change, and those who cannot change their minds cannot change anything."

–George Bernard Shaw

Beginning Your Day
What does this quote mean to me personally today?

_____

_____

How will I apply this quote today?

_____

_____

Who else needs to hear this quote today?

_____

_____

_____

At the End of Your Day
How did I apply this quote today?

_____

_____

What will I do differently going forward?

_____

_____

_____

"Life is a series of experiences, each one of which makes us bigger, even though sometimes it is hard to realize this. For the world was built to develop character, and we must learn that the setbacks and grieves which we endure help us in our marching onward."

–Henry Ford

Beginning Your Day
What does this quote mean to me personally today?

_____

_____

How will I apply this quote today?

_____

_____

Who else needs to hear this quote today?

_____

_____

_____

At the End of Your Day
How did I apply this quote today?

_____

_____

What will I do differently going forward?

_____

_____

_____

"If you aren't in the moment, you are either looking forward to uncertainty, or back to pain and regret."

–Jim Carrey

Beginning Your Day
What does this quote mean to me personally today?

_____
_____
_____

How will I apply this quote today?

_____
_____
_____

Who else needs to hear this quote today?

_____
_____
_____

At the End of Your Day
How did I apply this quote today?

_____
_____
_____

What will I do differently going forward?

_____
_____
_____

"I believe the world is one big family, and we need to help each other."

—Jet Li

Beginning Your Day
What does this quote mean to me personally today?

_____

_____

How will I apply this quote today?

_____

_____

Who else needs to hear this quote today?

_____

_____

_____

At the End of Your Day
How did I apply this quote today?

_____

_____

What will I do differently going forward?

_____

_____

_____

"Sometimes if you want to see a change for the better, you have to take things into your own hands."

–Clint Eastwood

Beginning Your Day
What does this quote mean to me personally today?

_____
_____
_____

How will I apply this quote today?

_____
_____
_____

Who else needs to hear this quote today?

_____
_____
_____

At the End of Your Day
How did I apply this quote today?

_____
_____
_____

What will I do differently going forward?

_____
_____
_____

"Nothing is impossible, the word itself says 'I'm possible'!"

—Audrey Hepburn

Beginning Your Day
What does this quote mean to me personally today?

_____

_____

How will I apply this quote today?

_____

_____

Who else needs to hear this quote today?

_____

_____

At the End of Your Day
How did I apply this quote today?

_____

_____

What will I do differently going forward?

_____

_____

_____

"The beginning is the most important part of the work."

–Plato

Beginning Your Day
What does this quote mean to me personally today?

_____

_____

How will I apply this quote today?

_____

_____

Who else needs to hear this quote today?

_____

_____

_____

At the End of Your Day
How did I apply this quote today?

_____

_____

What will I do differently going forward?

_____

_____

_____

"If your actions inspire others to dream more, learn more, do more and become more, you are a leader."

–John Quincy Adams

Beginning Your Day
What does this quote mean to me personally today?

_____

_____

How will I apply this quote today?

_____

_____

Who else needs to hear this quote today?

_____

_____

_____

At the End of Your Day
How did I apply this quote today?

_____

_____

What will I do differently going forward?

_____

_____

_____

"I think that music in itself is healing. It's an explosive expression of humanity. It's something we are all touched by. No matter what culture we're from, everyone loves music."

–Billy Joel

Beginning Your Day
What does this quote mean to me personally today?

_____

_____

_____

How will I apply this quote today?

_____

_____

_____

Who else needs to hear this quote today?

_____

_____

_____

At the End of Your Day
How did I apply this quote today?

_____

_____

_____

What will I do differently going forward?

_____

_____

_____

"I have found the paradox, that if you love until it hurts, there can be no more hurt, only more love."

–Mother Teresa

Beginning Your Day
What does this quote mean to me personally today?

_____

_____

How will I apply this quote today?

_____

_____

Who else needs to hear this quote today?

_____

_____

_____

At the End of Your Day
How did I apply this quote today?

_____

_____

What will I do differently going forward?

_____

_____

_____

" Integrity is everything. With it, you can weather all storms. Without it, even little things will derail you. Hold true to your commitments because relationships are either built or undone by them."

–Michael Stevenson

Beginning Your Day
What does this quote mean to me personally today?

_____
_____

How will I apply this quote today?

_____
_____

Who else needs to hear this quote today?

_____
_____
_____

At the End of Your Day
How did I apply this quote today?

_____
_____

What will I do differently going forward?

_____
_____
_____

"Mystery creates wonder and wonder is the basis of man's desire to understand."

–Neil Armstrong

Beginning Your Day
What does this quote mean to me personally today?

_____

_____

How will I apply this quote today?

_____

_____

Who else needs to hear this quote today?

_____

_____

_____

At the End of Your Day
How did I apply this quote today?

_____

_____

What will I do differently going forward?

_____

_____

_____

"In wisdom gathered over time I have found that every experience is a form of exploration."

—Ansel Adams

Beginning Your Day
What does this quote mean to me personally today?

_____

_____

How will I apply this quote today?

_____

_____

Who else needs to hear this quote today?

_____

_____

_____

At the End of Your Day
How did I apply this quote today?

_____

_____

What will I do differently going forward?

_____

_____

_____

"The size of your success is measured by the strength of your desire; the size of your dream; and how you handle disappointment along the way."

–Robert Kiyosaki

Beginning Your Day
What does this quote mean to me personally today?

_____

_____

How will I apply this quote today?

_____

_____

Who else needs to hear this quote today?

_____

_____

_____

At the End of Your Day
How did I apply this quote today?

_____

_____

What will I do differently going forward?

_____

_____

_____

"I am only one, but, I am one. I cannot do everything, but, I can do something, and I will not let what I cannot do interfere with what I can do."

–Edward Everett Hale

Beginning Your Day
What does this quote mean to me personally today?

_____

_____

_____

How will I apply this quote today?

_____

_____

_____

Who else needs to hear this quote today?

_____

_____

_____

At the End of Your Day
How did I apply this quote today?

_____

_____

_____

What will I do differently going forward?

_____

_____

_____

"You're going to go through tough times – that's life. But I say, 'Nothing happens to you, it happens for you.' See the positive in negative events."

–Joel Osteen

Beginning Your Day
What does this quote mean to me personally today?

_____

_____

How will I apply this quote today?

_____

_____

Who else needs to hear this quote today?

_____

_____

_____

At the End of Your Day
How did I apply this quote today?

_____

_____

What will I do differently going forward?

_____

_____

_____

"Never mistake motion for action."

–Ernest Hemingway

Beginning Your Day
What does this quote mean to me personally today?

_____

_____

How will I apply this quote today?

_____

_____

Who else needs to hear this quote today?

_____

_____

_____

At the End of Your Day
How did I apply this quote today?

_____

_____

What will I do differently going forward?

_____

_____

_____

"What is success? I think it is a mixture of having a flair for the thing that you are doing; knowing that it is not enough, that you have got to have hard work and a certain sense of purpose."

–Margaret Thatcher

Beginning Your Day
What does this quote mean to me personally today?

_____

_____

_____

How will I apply this quote today?

_____

_____

_____

Who else needs to hear this quote today?

_____

_____

_____

At the End of Your Day
How did I apply this quote today?

_____

_____

_____

What will I do differently going forward?

_____

_____

_____

"I don't believe in circumstances. The people who get on in this world are the people who get up and look for the circumstances they want, and, if they can't find them, make them."

—George Bernard Shaw

Beginning Your Day
What does this quote mean to me personally today?

_____

_____

How will I apply this quote today?

_____

_____

Who else needs to hear this quote today?

_____

_____

_____

At the End of Your Day
How did I apply this quote today?

_____

_____

What will I do differently going forward?

_____

_____

_____

"It is better to lead from behind and to put others in front, especially when you celebrate victory when nice things occur. You take the front line when there is danger. Then people will appreciate your leadership."

–Nelson Mandela

Beginning Your Day
What does this quote mean to me personally today?

_____

_____

How will I apply this quote today?

_____

_____

Who else needs to hear this quote today?

_____

_____

At the End of Your Day
How did I apply this quote today?

_____

_____

What will I do differently going forward?

_____

_____

_____

"We can learn something new anytime we believe we can."

–Virginia Satir

Beginning Your Day
What does this quote mean to me personally today?

_____
_____

How will I apply this quote today?

_____
_____

Who else needs to hear this quote today?

_____
_____
_____

At the End of Your Day
How did I apply this quote today?

_____
_____

What will I do differently going forward?

_____
_____
_____

"A wise man can learn more from a foolish question than a fool can learn from a wise answer."

–Bruce Lee

Beginning Your Day
What does this quote mean to me personally today?

_____

_____

How will I apply this quote today?

_____

_____

Who else needs to hear this quote today?

_____

_____

At the End of Your Day
How did I apply this quote today?

_____

_____

What will I do differently going forward?

_____

_____

_____

"Experience has shown, and a true philosophy will always show, that a vast, perhaps the larger portion of the truth arises from the seemingly irrelevant."

–Edgar Allan Poe

Beginning Your Day
What does this quote mean to me personally today?

_____

_____

How will I apply this quote today?

_____

_____

Who else needs to hear this quote today?

_____

_____

_____

At the End of Your Day
How did I apply this quote today?

_____

_____

What will I do differently going forward?

_____

_____

_____

"As long as we persevere and endure, we can get anything we want."

–Mike Tyson

Beginning Your Day
What does this quote mean to me personally today?

_____

_____

_____

How will I apply this quote today?

_____

_____

_____

Who else needs to hear this quote today?

_____

_____

_____

At the End of Your Day
How did I apply this quote today?

_____

_____

What will I do differently going forward?

_____

_____

_____

"To effectively communicate, we must realize that we are all different in the way we perceive the world and use this understanding as a guide to our communication with others."

–Tony Robbins

Beginning Your Day
What does this quote mean to me personally today?

_____

_____

How will I apply this quote today?

_____

_____

Who else needs to hear this quote today?

_____

_____

_____

At the End of Your Day
How did I apply this quote today?

_____

_____

What will I do differently going forward?

_____

_____

_____

"Don't find fault, find a remedy."

–Henry Ford

Beginning Your Day
What does this quote mean to me personally today?

_____

_____

How will I apply this quote today?

_____

_____

Who else needs to hear this quote today?

_____

_____

At the End of Your Day
How did I apply this quote today?

_____

_____

What will I do differently going forward?

_____

_____

_____

"Your smile will give you a positive countenance that will make people feel comfortable around you."

–Les Brown

Beginning Your Day
What does this quote mean to me personally today?

_____
_____
_____

How will I apply this quote today?

_____
_____
_____

Who else needs to hear this quote today?

_____
_____
_____

At the End of Your Day
How did I apply this quote today?

_____
_____
_____

What will I do differently going forward?

_____
_____
_____

"Do the one thing you think you cannot do. Fail at it. Try again. Do better the second time. The only people who never tumble are those who never mount the high wire. This is your moment. Own it."

–Oprah Winfrey

Beginning Your Day
What does this quote mean to me personally today?

_____

_____

How will I apply this quote today?

_____

_____

Who else needs to hear this quote today?

_____

_____

_____

At the End of Your Day
How did I apply this quote today?

_____

_____

What will I do differently going forward?

_____

_____

_____

"Open your eyes, look within. Are you satisfied with the life you're living?"

–Bob Marley

Beginning Your Day
What does this quote mean to me personally today?

_____
_____
_____

How will I apply this quote today?

_____
_____
_____

Who else needs to hear this quote today?

_____
_____
_____

At the End of Your Day
How did I apply this quote today?

_____
_____
_____

What will I do differently going forward?

_____
_____
_____

"Friends can help each other. A true friend is someone who lets you have total freedom to be yourself – and especially to feel. Or, not feel. Whatever you happen to be feeling at the moment is fine with them. That's what real love amounts to – letting a person be what he really is."

–Jim Morrison

Beginning Your Day
What does this quote mean to me personally today?

_____

_____

_____

How will I apply this quote today?

_____

_____

_____

Who else needs to hear this quote today?

_____

_____

_____

At the End of Your Day
How did I apply this quote today?

_____

_____

What will I do differently going forward?

_____

_____

_____

"Our greatest weakness lies in giving up. The most certain way to succeed is always to try just one more time."

–Thomas A. Edison

Beginning Your Day
What does this quote mean to me personally today?

_____

_____

How will I apply this quote today?

_____

_____

Who else needs to hear this quote today?

_____

_____

At the End of Your Day
How did I apply this quote today?

_____

_____

What will I do differently going forward?

_____

_____

_____

"Keep your face to the sunshine and you cannot see a shadow."

–Helen Keller

Beginning Your Day
What does this quote mean to me personally today?

_____

_____

_____

How will I apply this quote today?

_____

_____

_____

Who else needs to hear this quote today?

_____

_____

_____

At the End of Your Day
How did I apply this quote today?

_____

_____

What will I do differently going forward?

_____

_____

_____

"I have learned over the years that when one's mind is made up, that diminishes fear; knowing what must be done does away with fear."

–Rosa Parks

Beginning Your Day

What does this quote mean to me personally today?

_____

_____

How will I apply this quote today?

_____

_____

Who else needs to hear this quote today?

_____

_____

_____

At the End of Your Day

How did I apply this quote today?

_____

_____

What will I do differently going forward?

_____

_____

_____

"Always put your best self forward, and keep a smile on your face, because you never know when someone is being encouraged by, or falling in love with your smile."

–Kayla Moffett Stevenson

Beginning Your Day
What does this quote mean to me personally today?

_____

_____

_____

How will I apply this quote today?

_____

_____

_____

Who else needs to hear this quote today?

_____

_____

_____

At the End of Your Day
How did I apply this quote today?

_____

_____

_____

What will I do differently going forward?

_____

_____

_____

"If you can dream it, you can do it."

—Walt Disney

Beginning Your Day
What does this quote mean to me personally today?

_____

_____

_____

How will I apply this quote today?

_____

_____

_____

Who else needs to hear this quote today?

_____

_____

_____

At the End of Your Day
How did I apply this quote today?

_____

_____

_____

What will I do differently going forward?

_____

_____

_____

"The starting point of all achievement is desire."

–Napoleon Hill

Beginning Your Day
What does this quote mean to me personally today?

_____

_____

How will I apply this quote today?

_____

_____

Who else needs to hear this quote today?

_____

_____

At the End of Your Day
How did I apply this quote today?

_____

_____

What will I do differently going forward?

_____

_____

_____

"Any man who reads too much and uses his own brain too little falls into lazy habits of thinking."

–Albert Einstein

Beginning Your Day
What does this quote mean to me personally today?

_____

_____

How will I apply this quote today?

_____

_____

Who else needs to hear this quote today?

_____

_____

_____

At the End of Your Day
How did I apply this quote today?

_____

_____

What will I do differently going forward?

_____

_____

_____

"If you are the kind of person who is waiting for the 'right' thing to happen, you might wait for a long time. It's like waiting for all the traffic lights to be green for five miles before starting the trip."

–Robert Kiyosaki

Beginning Your Day
What does this quote mean to me personally today?

_____

_____

_____

How will I apply this quote today?

_____

_____

_____

Who else needs to hear this quote today?

_____

_____

_____

At the End of Your Day
How did I apply this quote today?

_____

_____

_____

What will I do differently going forward?

_____

_____

_____

"If we are not a little bit comfortable every day, we're not growing. All the good stuff is outside our comfort zone."

–Jack Canfield

Beginning Your Day
What does this quote mean to me personally today?

_____
_____

How will I apply this quote today?

_____
_____

Who else needs to hear this quote today?

_____
_____
_____

At the End of Your Day
How did I apply this quote today?

_____
_____

What will I do differently going forward?

_____
_____
_____

"The Constitution only gives people the right to pursue happiness. You have to catch it yourself."

–Benjamin Franklin

Beginning Your Day

What does this quote mean to me personally today?

_____

_____

How will I apply this quote today?

_____

_____

Who else needs to hear this quote today?

_____

_____

_____

At the End of Your Day

How did I apply this quote today?

_____

_____

What will I do differently going forward?

_____

_____

_____

"Darkness cannot drive out darkness; only light can do that. Hate cannot drive out hate; only love can do that."

–Martin Luther King, Jr.

Beginning Your Day
What does this quote mean to me personally today?

_____

_____

How will I apply this quote today?

_____

_____

Who else needs to hear this quote today?

_____

_____

_____

At the End of Your Day
How did I apply this quote today?

_____

_____

What will I do differently going forward?

_____

_____

_____

"When you practice gratefulness, there is a sense of respect toward others."

–Dalai Lama

Beginning Your Day
What does this quote mean to me personally today?

_____

_____

_____

How will I apply this quote today?

_____

_____

_____

Who else needs to hear this quote today?

_____

_____

_____

At the End of Your Day
How did I apply this quote today?

_____

_____

What will I do differently going forward?

_____

_____

_____

"Trust is the glue of life. It's the most essential ingredient in effective communication. It's the foundational principle that holds all relationships."

–Stephen Covey

Beginning Your Day
What does this quote mean to me personally today?

_____

_____

How will I apply this quote today?

_____

_____

Who else needs to hear this quote today?

_____

_____

_____

At the End of Your Day
How did I apply this quote today?

_____

_____

What will I do differently going forward?

_____

_____

_____

"I am always doing that which I cannot do, in order that I may learn how to do it."

–Pablo Picasso

Beginning Your Day
What does this quote mean to me personally today?

_____

_____

_____

How will I apply this quote today?

_____

_____

_____

Who else needs to hear this quote today?

_____

_____

_____

At the End of Your Day
How did I apply this quote today?

_____

_____

What will I do differently going forward?

_____

_____

_____

"I believe that through knowledge and discipline, financial peace is possible for all of us."

–Dave Ramsey

Beginning Your Day
What does this quote mean to me personally today?

_____

_____

How will I apply this quote today?

_____

_____

Who else needs to hear this quote today?

_____

_____

_____

At the End of Your Day
How did I apply this quote today?

_____

_____

What will I do differently going forward?

_____

_____

_____

"Hardships often prepare ordinary people for an extraordinary destiny."

–C.S. Lewis

Beginning Your Day
What does this quote mean to me personally today?

_____

_____

How will I apply this quote today?

_____

_____

Who else needs to hear this quote today?

_____

_____

_____

At the End of Your Day
How did I apply this quote today?

_____

_____

What will I do differently going forward?

_____

_____

_____

"I like to listen. I have learned a great deal from listening carefully. Most people never listen."

–Ernest Hemingway

Beginning Your Day
What does this quote mean to me personally today?

_____

_____

How will I apply this quote today?

_____

_____

Who else needs to hear this quote today?

_____

_____

_____

At the End of Your Day
How did I apply this quote today?

_____

_____

_____

What will I do differently going forward?

_____

_____

_____

"When I was 5 years old, my mother always told me that happiness was the key to life. When I went to school, they asked me what I wanted to be when I grew up. I wrote down 'happy'. They told me that I didn't understand the assignment, and I told them they didn't understand life."

–John Lennon

Beginning Your Day
What does this quote mean to me personally today?

_____

_____

_____

How will I apply this quote today?

_____

_____

_____

Who else needs to hear this quote today?

_____

_____

_____

At the End of Your Day
How did I apply this quote today?

_____

_____

_____

What will I do differently going forward?

_____

_____

_____

"Here's to the crazy ones, the misfits, the rebels, the troublemakers, the round pegs in the square holes, the ones who see things differently. They're not fond of rules. You can quote them, disagree with them, glorify or vilify them, but the only thing you can't do is ignore them because they change things... The ones who are crazy enough to think that they can change the world, are the ones who do." — *Steve Jobs*

Beginning Your Day
What does this quote mean to me personally today?

_____

_____

How will I apply this quote today?

_____

_____

Who else needs to hear this quote today?

_____

_____

_____

At the End of Your Day
How did I apply this quote today?

_____

_____

What will I do differently going forward?

_____

_____

_____

"You made it to the end! And now - what will your quote be? Speak it now, do it now, live it now and make it good!"

— Josephina

Beginning Your Day
What does this quote mean to me personally today?

_____

_____

How will I apply this quote today?

_____

_____

Who else needs to hear this quote today?

_____

_____

At the End of Your Day
How did I apply this quote today?

_____

_____

What will I do differently going forward?

_____

_____

_____

About The Author

Josephina lives works and plays in Roseville, California along with her husband, Steven and her many animals. She can't think of anything better than hanging out with her grandchildren!

She is a holistic weight loss coach and holds self-development workshops and seminars. Josephina loves to travel, and write children's books, and do anything creative. She invites you to visit her website and download your complimentary relaxing meditation so you can live your life better and better.

Visit her at www.FinaLouise.com

❤

29263737R00061

Printed in Great Britain
by Amazon